Edition

1

Physician's Style
Patient Note Writing

WHAT IS PHYSICIAN'S STYLE

PATIENT NOTE WRITING?

Simply put, physician style patient note writing addresses the art of writing patient note physician style. In other words it is about how doctors record their clinical encounter with their patient starting from first time of meeting the patient to the last time the patient is seen.

This book shows the reader how to write a physician style, consistent standard patient note.

As a medical doctor, your patient note is a major part of your evidence for services provided to your patient and your reference for continuation of care. You must write it well.

Always Keep Clinical Records

Physician's Style – Patient Note Writing

Our patients depend on us for their health.

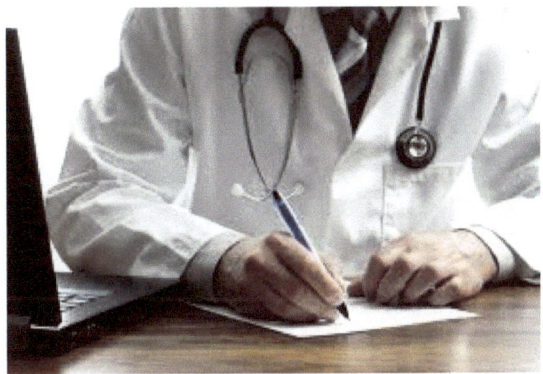

A physician's note is part of that care and must be taken seriously.

The medical doctor must know how to write a concise patient note for the benefit of his or her patient, facility and the law.

Table of Contents

Chapter

1

Keys to Writing a Professional Patient Note

This book is intended to guide a physician to write an accurate and concise patient note that meets all standards of practice.

A s a physician, your patient note is your written tool of communication to any authorized care giver in your multi-disciplinary team, who may come in contact with or render any form of care to your patient.

In this book, it is assumed that the reader already knows how to obtain patient history, how to perform a physical exam and what is required for workup and management.

What is a Patient Note?

Whenever a patient contacts a physician for any health concern, there are three major encounters that occur between the doctor and his/ her patient.

1.   Initial contact:

This is when the patient and the doctor make the first contact. At this stage, the doctor interviews the patient in order to figure out what is bothering the patient. The doctor also documents the findings from the history and initial examination of the patient in a standard professional systematic manner.

2.   Progress of Care:

Next, as care is rendered, the patient is re-evaluated and all findings are systematically recorded including new findings, improvements, changes to treatment.

3. Discharge:

At discharge, the patient is re-evaluated and all findings and recommendations are documented as discharge notes.

You use the Patient Note to express your patient interviews, observations, impressions, treatments and outcomes of the management you provide.

More importantly, your Patient Note is a legal documentation of the care you rendered your patient at your facility or elsewhere, which is admissible in a court of law in all cases of litigation or malpractice cases.

It is therefore of paramount importance that you write a concise, legible, brief patient note at all times and in all patient encounters. That means that you, the doctor, have the obligation to write an accurate patient note at all times.

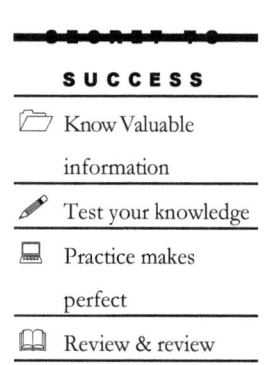

SUCCESS

🗁 Know Valuable
information

✏ Test your knowledge

💻 Practice makes
perfect

📖 Review & review

In order to write a Patient Note, the first thing to consider is to know how to write an inclusive, short or brief, clear patient note that communicates pertinent information to the reader.

The following are things that you must know very well in order to be able to accurately write a patient note:

1. Know short forms of medical statements and abbreviations, especially those used at your facility.

For example,

Doctor Adam writes:

The patient's name is Mrs. Jones. She is 25 years old. She came into the clinic today complaining of right lower abdominal pains which started bothering her since two months ago. She said that her menstrual periods have been regular but the last two months her periods have been scanty.

Doctor Bradley writes:

Mrs. Jones, 25 yo F, c/o RLQ pains since 2 months. LMP-2 weeks ago, regular, <1 pad/day last 2 consecutive months.

From these two examples, Doctor Bradley's note is brief compared to that of Doctor Adam, with the same information.

Short forms are allowed but they must be within the approved standard for all doctors or for your facility, so that all clinicians can understand the intended communication.

2. Know disease symptoms and treatments.

    With this knowledge, you will be able to have a sound differential diagnosis in order to arrive at the correct workups and medical diagnosis.

    Common patient problems presented at outpatient clinics are:

    - Headache

    - Pain

    - Fever/Flu

    - HTN

    - Diarrhea

    - Weight gain

    - Weight loss

    - Stroke

    - DM

    - Pregnancy

    - Bleeding

    - Trauma

How to avoid costly mistakes

Avoiding costly mistakes is a goal that every physician, practicing or in training should seek.

You avoid mistakes by taking the time to learn your profession properly so that you have the tool of the trade.

You also need to be thorough and always put yourself in the place of others whenever you do things.

Write clearly and legibly. For example, how do you feel if you are a nurse and cannot read a doctor's patient note? What time costs can that amount to?

What danger does this pose to your patient if the information in your patient note misleads the nurse to give the wrong medication (medication errors) or care? Suppose the nurse turns and walks a patient that you placed on bed rest because she/he could not read your writing? Or, what if your nurse administers a wrong dose of a drug with extremely narrow therapeutic index? Think about that.

If your nurse cannot understand your writing or your orders, she/ he can make a dangerous mistake while caring for your patient.

Remember you have 15 minutes to collect patient information

Always be aware of time.

A physician has many patients waiting at the office or for an appointment.

You must always consider the time factor while collecting all patient data and when writing patient note.

Organize your time for optimum efficiency.

You should organize your patient note in a consistent order to avoid missing out important information.

How to Organize Your Patient Note

The patient note has certain parts that must be included when written.

The following parts are used by practicing physicians:

1. History

2. Physical Examination

3. Differential Diagnosis

4. Diagnostic Workup

5. Diagnosis

6. Management

The following parts are required to pass the USMLE Step 1 CS exam:

1. History

2. Physical Exam

3. Differential Diagnosis

4. Diagnostic Workup

INITIAL ENCOUNTER

1. History

What should be included in patient history?

- Demographic information – name, sex, age, allergies, work type, medications

- Chief Complaint, CC

- History of present illness, HPI

- Review of systems, ROS – general health status of all systems. Pay attention to negative complaints and the system involved.

- Past medical history, PMH – includes hospitalizations, surgeries, medical conditions, birth history.

- Social history, SH – does your patient drink alcohol, smoke or use recreational (illicit) drugs? What is his/ her sexual life like? Does he or she have more than one sexual partner? Is he or she sexually active and does he or she have sex with both men and women?

- Family history, FH – are parents alive or dead, cause of death or illness, children alive and well, spouse and support systems.

2. Physical Examination

Write your impression about the outward appearance of your patient. Is he or she in active distress or not?

Vital signs – record and assess vital signs

HEENT – head, eyes, ears, nose and throat. Write any problems or no problems here.

Neck – check for enlarged lymph nodes and other abnormalities and record your findings.

Chest – listen to your patient's chest and record your findings.

Heart – listen to the heart and record.

Abdomen – (a) visually observe the abdomen for shape, swellings, discolorations, peristalsis, (b) listen through the four quadrants of the abdomen for peristalsis and other sounds, (c) perform a systemic all abdominal palpation and record your findings.

Skin – this is a valuable clinical examination because some diseases can present with skin symptoms. It is mandatory in skin disease.

Chapter

3

HANDWRITING

All about your handwriting doc

Hand Writing

The look and feel of your patient note depends upon your handwriting. If you have a poor, illegible handwriting, do yourself and your patient a favor. Type your patient note or print all letters and characters in all your documentations. You definitely do not want nor need an illegible note that is misleading because that can be dangerous to your patient's health and can easily land you in court if any errors are made along any line in your patient care.

Avoid Errors

To avoid errors, simply review your notes and make corrections. Make sure you are clear and that someone else can read what you wrote.

Always write in black ink because there are people who may be color blind reading your patient note at some point and you want all information entered to be visible.

Concise & Brevity Are Key

In this book, you will learn how to be brief and concise in your patient note writing. This is the key to writing a winning patient note.

Using the Brief
Insert brief acronyms and abbreviations in your patient note to inform and save time

Being concise and brief means writing your note to the point meant, no extra unnecessary distracting information required. Write to the point without omitting relevant information but without including irrelevant information that can only distract or confuse your reader from the objective of your note.

To do this, you need to learn the language of medicine using common statements and abbreviations that your peers and other members of your multi-disciplinary team can understand. The goal is to keep everything clear and short.

Common Medical Acronyms and Abbreviations

It is permissible to use short forms of medical words or acronyms to express information in your patient note. Just make sure the abbreviations are the ones approved by your facility and practice.

For the USMLE, you can find these abbreviations at the USMLE website.

Below are examples of some permissible abbreviations that can be used in most United States hospitals, healthcare facilities and practice:

Sample Common Abbreviations that can be used for writing the Patient Note

Note: There is no need to use abbreviations on the patient note if you are in doubt about the correct abbreviation. Write the word or phrase out completely when in doubt.

yo .... year-old

M .... male
F .... female
b ....black
w............. white
L ....left
R............ right
hx ....history
h/o ....history of
c/o ....complaining of
Ø ....without or no
+........... positive
- ....negative

abd .... Abdomen

ABG......... arterial blood gas

am...............morning

ad lib........................at discretion

AIDS............. acquired immune deficiency syndrome

AP .... antero-posterior

AK....................above knee

BUN .... blood urea nitrogen

CABG............... coronary artery bypass grafting

CAD ....coronary artery disease

CBC.................. complete blood count

CCU.................. cardiac care unit

CHF .... congestive heart failure

Cig .... cigarettes

COPD........................... chronic obstructive pulmonary disease

CPR............................. cardiopulmonary resuscitation

Chapter

4

Types of Patient Note for physicians

There are various types of patient note writing commonly used in most hospitals, healthcare facilities and medical practices.

The patient note can be categorized by brevity as:

1. Narrative Style. This type involves writing the patient note in a narrative way, in other words, you the doctor tell your story about your patient encounter.

2. Telegraphic Style. This type of note writing is presented in a "bullet" format, using short phrases or incomplete sentences to convey information.

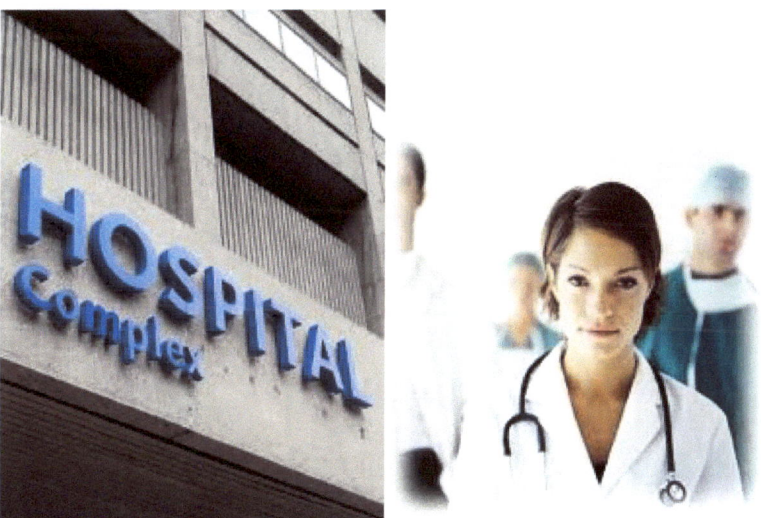

**Samples of part
patient note with
narrative and
bullet style**

Narrative Style:

25 yo F c/o mild chest pain. Symptoms started 2 hrs. ago after a fatty meal. Pain is mid chest, burning, no radiation. Denies SOB, nausea and diaphoresis. Has mild pain now. Worse with meals and after lying down. Improves with OTC antacids treatment. No prior hx. Has hx of HTN and depression. On daily antihypertensive meds. Not on antipsychotic now. Mother with NIDDM, HTN and high cholesterol. Only child. Single, lives alone, nursing student.

Telegraphic Style:

- 25 yo F,

- CC – Chest pain x 2 hrs

- HPI – Started after fatty meal

- _ - nausea

- _ - SOB

- _ -diaphoresis

- _ Denies similar past episodes

- _ Pain better with antacids.

- PMH _ HTN, No DM. Daily antihypertensive. No antipsychotics now.

- FSH - Only child, lives alone. Student. Mother-NIDDM, HTN, ↑cholesterol.

Chapter

5

Parts of Patient Note:

1. History-

The patient history is the information gathered from the patient during doctor-patient interview.

This information should be documented systematically in the patient note as follows:

- Demographics – name of patient, age, sex, known allergies, Advanced Directive(CODE Status)

- CC – chief complaints

- HPI – history of present illness

- PMSH – past medical & surgical history

- FSH – family & social history

2. Physical Examination

This part of your patient note should contain all your findings during physical examination of your patient.

You should start your physical exam systematically from head to toe, starting first with

- ✓ visual inspection

- ✓ auscultation

- ✓ percussion

✓ palpation

Record accordingly as follows:

- General observation– any obvious distress, appearance and posture

- skin – discolorations, bruises, skin tags, lesions

- Head & Neck - check for swelling and obvious abnormalities, eyes for sight, ears for hearing, mouth for lesions

- Chest – deformity, lung & heart sounds, crepitus, size, shape

- Abdomen – distention, bowel sounds, masses

- Upper Limbs – contractures, size, length, anatomical position, use, ROM, deformity, nails, clubbing

- Lower Limbs - contractures, size, length, anatomical position, use, ROM, deformity, nails, clubbing

- Musculoskeletal – contractures, disuse, use, ambulation

- Neurological – all neurological tests pertinent to your patient's case.

3. Differential Diagnosis

Once you conclude on an impression which is the diagnosis, you then need to differentiate that diagnosis from other diseases with similar symptoms before your workup.

For example:

A patient with: CC - headache.

What is your differential diagnosis? { Intracranial Mass, Migraine, Tension Headaches, Pseudo tumor Cerebri, Cluster Headaches, Temporal Arteritis, or Sinusitis}

What workup do you plan to use to help this patient? Start by checking the CBC, ESR, CT & MRI of head and brain respectively, Temporal artery biopsy, sinus CT scan. If patient has fever, do a blood culture and sensitivity as well.

4. Diagnosis

Knowing what your patient has is most important to arriving at the correct diagnosis, which is affected by your differential diagnosis and your workup plan. You can arrive at a medical diagnosis after a good differential diagnosis and a thorough workup.

You should learn how to gather information from your patient in a systematic manner and use that information and your knowledge about various diseases to arrive at your medical diagnosis.

The best thing to do is to develop, write down your own preferred practice note on patient history gathering technic, and know differential diagnosis for illnesses and the workup for each case. Stick with that in all your cases. You'll see that after a while it becomes a routine and easy to remember.

Always start your physical assessments in a consistent fashion such as from the head to toe direction.

Tips on systematic consistent physical exam

Say you have a patient to perform a physical exam on:

First perform a general visual overview from head to toe (review of systems) – head, check for swellings, bruises, discoloration, heat, cold, lymph node enlargements, throat swelling etc.

Next check the neck, distended jugular vein, skin, lymph nodes, and vein distention.

The Chest is next, check for shape (barrel shaped or WNL), lumps, discoloration.

The abdomen is checked for visual peristaltic movements of bowel, distention and shape.

Extremities are checked for any visually observable contractures, signs of possible disuse of limb, length, alignment, position and activity.

The next step is to go back and check all the systems more thoroughly in the same sequence of head-neck-chest-abdomen-extremities or neurological.

Head – palpate for deformity, trauma, lumps, and enlarged lymph nodes. Perform a fundoscopy to check eyes, check sclera for any injection or redness, check the nose, ears for abnormality.

Neck – Check for jugular vein distension, palpate for swellings, masses or enlarged lymph nodes.

Chest – listen for breath sounds (vesicular, crepitation, rhonchi), heart sounds (1&2, murmurs, rhythm, strength), palpate for abnormal masses, percuss for hollow sounds.

Abdomen – Shape (flat, distension, and deformity); listen for bowel sounds all four quadrants, percuss for abdominal echoes, palpate for masses (size, consistency, mobility).

Extremities – Upper and lower extremities. Check for length, alignment, movement, contractures, swellings (edema or tumor), ulcers, neurological abnormalities.

How to generate a work-up plan

To generate a work up, you must arrive at the correct differential diagnosis.

You can only arrive at a correct differential diagnosis if you are aware of all the diseases that present with similar symptoms as the case you have at hand.

Then, you choose the most likely, common, deadly of the lot.

By doing so, you help rule out the disease that may cause more harm to your patient.

Note

You can write a compelling note if you are thorough and consistent

Chapter

6

Time Management

Keeping a template handy can save you time. This is of course my personal experience. We must remember that each patient is unique and requires specific history, work-up and management which can of course be added or removed from the template.

What I do is that each day, I map out my hours and assign a schedule of how to spend each minute. It may not work for everyone, but it does work for me. That way, I can finish my daily work load and make sure that none of my patients waits longer than necessary at the office.

How to Save Time in the Future

When you save your note template with your changes, it will be easier to create documents in the future. To customize this note:

1. Insert your patient information in place of the saved sample and in short order your current patient information will be ready.

2. Save your template preferably on a computer. However, you can save a hard copy as a reference to writing.

   That way you don't have to start over writing each time from scratch.

Save a template to save time in future.

Time is expensive to a functioning doctor. Use your time wisely.

Below is a sample patient note template form:

Patient Name: _____ Date: _____

Sex: _____ Age: _____ DOB: _____

SSN: _____ Hospital #: _____

Next of Kin: _____ Contact: _____

Home Address: _____

_____

_____

Telephone   #:   _____   email:

_____

Allergies: _____ DNR: ☐

History

Chief Complaint(CC)
History of present illness(HPI)
Past Medical History(PMH)
Family History(FH)
Review of Systems(ROS)

Physical Examination

- General Inspection and overview
- Palpation
- Percussion
- Auscultation

Systems that must be examined:
Head & neck
Chest
Abdomen
Neurological

Differential Diagnosis

Work up

Labs

Diagnosis

Management

Chapter
7

Fix errors in your patient note

How to Change errors in your patient note

To change errors in your note, simply draw one clean straight line once across the error, initial below or on top of your line and continue to write-in the correct intended word or sentence.

JKJ 02/17/11

For example: ~~pt L arm...~~   pt R arm...

How to create a clear note

To create a clear patient note:

- Write legibly so that no one in your medical team may have any problem understanding your communication.

- Use standard writing supplies approved by your facility or office.

- Clearly delete errors if writing online or draw a line across your errors followed by your initials and date as explained above if your note is on paper, replacing them with corrections.

Chapter

8

More Patient Note Tips

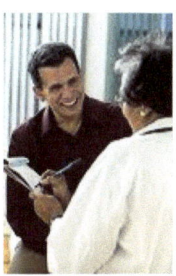

Patients are sick and need to be seen as soon as possible. Watch your time so that you don't keep others waiting for long periods.

Build trust on each encounter so that the patient will give you the information that you are seeking.

Know your medical facts so that you can quickly differentiate between diseases and arrive at an accurate diagnosis and treatment.

Chapter

9

PATIENT PROGRESS NOTE

How is the patient doing with your treatment?

Progress Notes

The progress note is a follow up note that you write daily as you follow the progress of your patient with management.

Usually the progress note is brief and can be about one paragraph in length. However, if there are new developments with your patient and his or her care, you must include your findings in your daily progress note.

Note main problems that the patient has and what has been done and the outcome of intervention. It is not necessary to re-write none pertinent information as was recorded in the initial history.

You also can state new medications and cancellations that you may order as well as discharge notices in the progress note.

Sample Progress Note:

01/07/12

Ms. Johnson states that her pain is at a 5 on a scale of 10 for pain. She claims to tolerate walking better today than yesterday.

Rx: Discontinue IV Morphine.

Tylenol 325 mg bd q 12 h

Signed

Physician, MD

Chapter

10

TIME for DISCHARGE

Discharge Notes

Use discharge notes to communicate your care to the discharge nurse, other team members and to new facilities that the patient may be going to in order to further treatment.

Your discharge note should contain the summary of care given, new orders for home or referrals for consultation and other facilities.

Chapter

11

FACTS ABOUT DOCUMENTATION

Documentation is one of the most important parts of your work as physician.

The patient note is a written documentation of your clinical encounter with your patient. It is your evidence that you actually cared for your patient. Therefore close attention must be paid when documenting all encounters with patients.

The note you write and document is your legal evidence for care given and is usually used in cases of litigation in court.

It is important to start practicing writing concise patient note with documentation of what was done. First, always write date and time for each encounter or treatment rendered. Next write subjective and objective findings before and after every encounter or procedure. Then, enter the patient's response to treatments and any follow up required. Do not forget to include all labs ordered and medication.

Patient Note is not the only documentation related to your patient. For instance, nurses, social workers, consultants and other multi-disciplinary team members all have their own respective ways of documenting their care of the same patient.

Always note the date and time of your encounter in any clinical documentation you record, because if something happens, say you are to testify in court, it is hard to accurately remember what happened and when. Your note will have the information if you only had spent a few seconds and recorded it.

ACKNOWLEDGEMENTS

I am extremely grateful to my parents who played a huge role in educating and making me who I am today.

Thanks to my family and friends who stood by me through my journey.